Family Medical Planning

Amy Rose Herrick, ChFC

For Randy,

Thank you for helping me in so many different ways every day.

Table of Contents

Introduction

Why would I write a whole book about multi-generational medical planning issues?

I have seen the real life results of those who planned for a medical emergency in advance and the tragic results of those who have not.

In every family, no matter who you define as your family, what affects one family member affects all family members at different levels.

For the small business owner your employees are a unique second family. Whatever affects your employee family affects your business day to day operations and your customer or sales retention. All of these are directly tied to your bottom line. Knowing how to protect your business cash flow from a catastrophic medical event for you or a key employee is a vital part of your ongoing operational plans that is too often ignored until a crisis occurs, and then it is too late to change your results.

This book is designed for families at any age or stage of life to enable you to understand and discuss difficult situations you may face some day. Perhaps you have already experienced personally how just one major medical crisis can impact three or more generations. I have.

In this book you will learn what you need to know about various insurance product options and important legal documents before they are needed.

This easy to read general reference tool was written without a lot of technical terms or the over use of abbreviated initials intentionally. Technical terms and jumbles of capital letters you don't recognize instantly are distracting. I avoided using them whenever possible for your benefit.

This resource will guide you in many useful ways to customize a well thought out plan of action for your family before a medical crisis occurs.

At the end of the book I have included a resource checklist for your convenience. You may want to take a moment to make notes there after reading each chapter.

Amy Rose Herrick, ChFC
Christiansted, U.S. Virgin Islands
February, 2015

Chapter One:
Why is a Medical Event a Family Problem?

Former First Lady Rosalyn Carter is credited with these insightful words at
http://www.alzheimersreadingroom.com/2009/11/quote-of-day-caregivers.html

> *There are only four kinds of people in the world -*
> *Those who have been caregivers,*
> *Those who currently are caregivers,*
> *Those who will be caregivers,*
> *And those who will need caregivers.*

It does not matter how young or old you are when a medical crisis occurs.

Your situation affects everyone around you.

All available resources in your family will be diverted to the one in need.

Even if you are not the person who is ill or injured, you may be required to make a long term investment of your time and labors to help out.

You may be responsible for scheduling doctors' appointments, surgical procedures or other treatments. You may need to accompany the person requiring medical attention.

You may be required to pay large lump sums of money upfront or agree to long term installment payments to pay off the staggering costs of your family member's treatment.

You may need to be available for emotional support. Perhaps you will be a strong shoulder to cry on. Maybe you will just sit, holding a hand, listening to the struggles your family member is enduring.

If you hold the Medical Power of Attorney (MPOA) of a loved one you may be required to make treatment decisions for a loved one who is unable to make decisions on his or her own.

If you hold the Financial Power of Attorney (POA) of a loved one you may be required to make some difficult financial decisions that will have long term effects regarding income, income taxes and asset liquidations.

Some readers will juggle all these challenging roles simultaneously.

With a little forethought you can mitigate much of the financial, procedural, emotional and time consuming stressors associated with these life events before they happen to you and your family.

Susan's Story

"Emily, I'm so grateful for all the help you have given me, and paying for lunch out today, too," says Susan to her long-time friend. "The offer of a loan is appreciated, and you are so sweet to offer it to us. Even with the money my folks have given us we will still lose our home in the next few weeks."

Emily looks stunned. She apparently has no idea Susan's situation was this bad.

"We have been selling about everything extra we have. We've had four garage sales already, you know. I sold some things on eBay and we sold our second car several months ago. We have let go of so much trying to bring in some type of income for us.

"With the foreclosure costs looming, I doubt we will see one cent of the house sale proceeds. Our credit is ruined with all the missed or late payments already piled up.

"Even if someone agreed to loan us more, we can't afford the payments with me not working. Steve is working overtime when he can, and doing odd jobs when they come up. But I also need him at home spending time with the boys like he used to before all this happened. He is exhausted most of the time and worried about how to pay the next past due notice. Some days I try not to let him see the mail.

"I am mostly worried about finding a new place to live. And moving costs money that we just don't have. I spent every dime of my savings and retirement funds long ago. We want to keep the boys in the same school district with their friends, but that looks unlikely with the costs of rental housing nearby. My parents downsized to a small two bedroom house a few years ago. It's just too tiny for all of us to live in even though they offered to enclose the garage to create more living space. Besides, it is so far away from here; Steve would have to commute on top of everything else."

Emily can only listen as the whole picture came pouring out of Susan, who is doing her best to remain composed.

"I know it sounds stupid now," Susan continues, "but in an attempt to make minimum payments, keep the utilities on, and some food on the table while I tried to get well, I took credit card cash advances until they were maxed out. I even maxed out one of my parents' cards they gave me. I am so ashamed that on top of all the money they have already given us, Mom is also making those payments for me right now so her credit is not ruined, too,.

"My dad said he will just work a little longer. I feel awful about that, too. He was looking forward to retiring soon. They were planning on buying a new car for Mom's birthday. Now they can't afford it because of the cash they've spent on me."

Susan takes another slow, deep breath and pushes her salad around on the plate in front of her with a fork. "Now the doctors are telling me that I should stay off of work for at least another six months to finish my treatment and recover my strength after the surgeries and physical therapy. I have at least six more months of this!

"I've got to be realistic about working again, too. I hope I have a job to go back to someday. I was in and out on sick leave over the period of almost a year altogether with this. If I have to add another six months before being eligible for re-employment with the company, I don't know if there will be a job when I am ready to go back. I have heard from a co-worker that my company is struggling with recent changes in the marketplace and the possibility of a job still existing there looks pretty grim even if I am well enough to get back into my sales position before the end of the year. It's a small company and they do not have the luxury of a big corporation behind them to float it for a while if needed financially."

Emily just nods and murmurs encouragement.

Susan, obviously very troubled, wipes away a silent tear and then continues, "With all the problems in front of me I know that I need to talk to an attorney about filing bankruptcy. I don't want to do it. Do you think if I file bankruptcy I will lose my team of doctors? I am already in debt to them and owe them thousands of dollars. Will they stop seeing me? Where would I go? A few months ago I thought having a good job, savings and some health insurance was enough, but now I know it isn't. I'm scared. What do I do now?"

Emily tries to respond and be helpful, but everything she can think of feels like old clichés that don't apply here. Emily hears herself trying to sound positive, saying things she has heard before: "I know things will get better soon. For now, just focus on getting well." Her mind is racing. She becomes increasingly concerned about her own family situation. What if her family's medical circumstances ever mirrored Susan's? What would she do differently? What could she do differently?

Sitting there with a knot in her stomach Emily knows nothing short of a miracle can save her friend from her next impending financial disaster.

Susan is losing almost everything she worked so hard for. At this point, it's like being strapped into a gigantic financial roller coaster. The car she is trapped in is rapidly going only downhill at increasing speeds. She is being twisted and jerked in new terrifying directions with every turn of the wheels on the precarious tracks. She can't even see a point to focus on where this unnerving ride will end. Susan keeps hanging on for dear life. She is waiting for her surreal ride to finally come to a screeching halt. If she could just stop somewhere, just get this to stop anywhere but where she is right now it would have to be an improvement. All she wants deep inside is to finally be able to stand on solid ground again. She needs some part of the comfortable life she once knew to return to normal.

Although bankruptcy may be the only recourse left for Susan and her family, even this does not solve all the problems. In fact, bankruptcy often creates new problems.

What Susan is facing is not uncommon. Whether it is an accident or an illness, the financial results can be the same. Many of these individuals and families have inadequate savings, investments, and insurance benefits. Many who are insured are still financially devastated.

If Susan had a crystal ball a few months or years earlier, do you think she would have made changes in her lifestyle that included setting aside some of her income for more comprehensive insurance and estate planning?

Most of us have been told to build an emergency savings cushion. The ideal primary accumulation vehicles in most households would be liquid, nonfluctuating accounts such as savings accounts, money markets or short duration CDs for reserves totaling three to six months of gross income. If you are a small business owner or self-employed, you may need to have larger liquid cash reserves to pay ongoing operating expenses for similar time periods.

Savings is just the tip of the iceberg on what you need to know.

You need to have documents and plans in place to avoid Susan's story happening to you.

In Susan's story, three generations were impacted by just one illness. The family will likely never recover financially from the overall effects. Here are some of the consequences of Susan and her family having inadequate planning for catastrophic medical events:

• Susan and Steve's once excellent credit has been ruined. This makes borrowing even for a car in the future more expensive. When they can qualify to borrow again it will at much higher interest rates for years after the bankruptcy.

• The kids' college funds have been eliminated.

• Vacations, summer camp, cable TV extras and other family leisure activities they enjoyed in the past cannot be repeated for a long time. There is no extra money for unnecessary or leisure activities with outstanding past due bills to pay.

• Susan's parents' retirement must be delayed for several years as they financially help Susan and her family. They will work longer to rebuild their own decimated emergency savings.

• Susan's parents are postponing buying anything that is not absolutely essential.

• Susan's parents' delayed retirement is also heavily dependent on not experiencing a similar medical crisis of their own over the next several years.

• Any hope of retirement for Susan and Steve has been destroyed.

Statistics Are Ugly

Here are some startling research results that may motivate you to act to protect your family, resources and assets so that you do not repeat Susan's story:

• 76% of Americans are living paycheck to paycheck.
http://money.cnn.com/2013/06/24/pf/emergency-savings

• According to the Federal Reserve, 44% of U.S. families spend more than they earn.
Federal Reserve Board, Survey of Consumer Finances 2004
Parade Magazine, Is the American Dream Still Possible?, April 23, 2006

• Most American workers can't afford to become disabled; over 70% of working Americans do not have enough savings to meet short-term emergencies.
National Investment Watch Survey, A.G. Edwards Inc. 2004

• Over 50% of the workforce has no private pension coverage and a third have no retirement savings. *Social Security Administration, Fact Sheet 2007*

• Disability causes nearly 50% of all mortgage foreclosures; 2% are caused by death. *Health Affairs, The Policy Journal of the Health Sphere, 2 February 2005*

• In one study three quarters of the individuals who filed for medical bankruptcy had health insurance. http://www.amjmed.com/article/S0002-9343(09)00404-5/abstract

• Using identical definitions in 2001 and 2007, the share of bankruptcies attributable to medical problems rose by 49.6%. http://www.amjmed.com/article/S0002-9343(09)00404-5/abstract

• While many people think that disabilities are typically caused by freak accidents, the majority of long-term absences are due to back injuries and illnesses such as cancer and heart disease. *Council for Disability Awareness, Long-Term Disability Claims Review, 2007*

• 498 Americans became disabled in the last 10 minutes. *National Safety Council, Injury Facts 2008 Ed.*

• An illness or accident will keep 1 in 5 workers out of work for at least a year before the age of 65. *Life and Health Insurance Foundation for Education, November 2005*

• One in 7 workers can expect to be disabled for five years or more before retirement. *"Commissioners Disability Table, 1998," Health Insurance Association of America, the New York Times, February 2000*

• Over 51 million Americans are classified as disabled, representing 18% of the population. *U.S. Census Bureau, Public Information Office, November 2008*

$23,215 A Year and Rising

Milliman, a leading national insurance actuarial and product development firm reported in 2014 that a "typical" insured family of four in the U.S. will spend $23,215 on medical care. This figure was compiled using data only for an average employer sponsored plan. On average, employers pick up 58% of this cost, but that still leaves a lot of uncovered costs for the average family to bear.

For those outside of the study parameters who do not have employer-sponsored coverage, the average costs are not available and could easily be higher without a group type network or other discounts available.

Medical costs have increased annually for more than a decade. Is it reasonable to hope that the inflationary trend will decrease? Whether single or with a family, planning for increases in health care costs is a necessity.

It really is all about money (and TIME) and *time really is money*.

Expenses for normal everyday life will not simply go away. What happens in an emergency? The bills do not pay themselves, and don't forget — there are the "crisis" figures, too. This is money that you must have for additional expenses in times of need. Consider the following:

- You need to continue paying your mortgage or rent payments to retain a place to live.

- You need to pay for essential utilities such as electricity, water, phone, gas, etc. for comfort and healing.

- You must buy food and beverages to survive.

- After insurance pays their portion, how much more is needed for your portion including co-pays and deductibles?

- You need to determine and budget a separate dollar figure for expected non-covered treatment expenses and home modifications.

- You need to allow room in your budget for increased transportation costs.

Expenses can escalate even faster if a family member must take unpaid time off work to help with medical treatments or transportation to and from appointments.

Just getting a patient from home, into the building from the parking lot, into the provider's office and then doing it all again in reverse is very time consuming, even for short office visits.

If prescriptions need filled or new medical devices need fitted, ordered and purchased, even more driving and waiting time is required.

It is very common for a sick or injured person needing ongoing care to be restricted from driving during the healing process for an indefinite period of time.

For some patients the illness or injury triggers an additional emotionally upsetting change in their lifestyle. They may become physically or mentally unable to drive as a result of a medical condition.

Some patients may require the revocation of their driver's license in order to insure the wellbeing of themselves as well as others. This new lifestyle change for everyone is an emotionally charged experience for all involved.

Losing another piece of their independence can be very hard for some patients to deal with.

This is a significant lifestyle change eliminating prior day to day freedoms they have often taken for granted. Most people in this situation have been driving for decades prior to this occurrence. Now even routine trips to the grocery store, church services or for a simple haircut can become a scheduling ordeal for the driver/chauffeur.

Don't forget the assisting family member is impacted heavily too. Will an assisting family member's lost wages and vehicle operating expenses need funded? How will they be financially compensated fairly for their time and efforts?

In order to retain employment some people use the family medical leave act that is available to employees who need to assist family members. This benefit will protect their employment, but in most instances it is unpaid leave. It is not an option available to every worker depending on the size of the employer. Consult with your Human Resources Department for help in understanding your company policy in this area.

A disability may require the spouse or adult child caregiver to spend less time at work. This could lead to a reduction of family income. The financial implications affect everyone, making it a multi-generational family planning issue.

An often neglected consideration is the affected employers. They have businesses to run. How long can they afford to keep ill or injured employees at a reduced schedule or hold a position vacant? Do they lose income when employees take medical leave?

There is a great deal to consider if you become disabled:

- Where will your income come from?

- Do you own a personal disability insurance plan?

- Does your employer have a short or long term disability insurance plan for employees via payroll deduction?

- Income replacement plans will usually replace no more than 60 to 70% of your pre-disability income. If your expenses stay the same or increase at the same time where will the rest of your income requirements come from?

- If you are paying the premiums, the benefits are usually not included in your taxable income when received.

• If your employer is paying the premium, the benefits usually are taxable income when received.

• When do your benefits start? Like a payroll check, you must "earn the benefit" before it is paid.

• If you have a 90-day waiting period, you probably won't see the first check until 120 to 150 days after your disability date. How will you pay your bills during that four to five month lag time?

• What is the maximum number of payments you could expect or at what age will they cease?

Chapter Two:
Seven Steps to Take Now to Protect Your Family Assets

How can you avoid being a financially devastated statistic like Susan? Simple: here is a seven-part income and asset protection solution designed to enable you to control your out-of-pocket costs, limit your overall financial exposure, reduce your income taxes, provide an income stream in the event of illness or injury, and secure real peace of mind for yourself, your family, and your household.

Step One:
Various Health Plans

If you do not have a good group health plan option, secure a Qualified Health Savings Account (HSA) that pays 100% of covered expenses after the deductible is met.

In 2015, this could limit your covered medical expense exposure as a "single person" to a maximum of $3,350 (adjusted annually), or for a family an annual covered expense maximum of only $6,650 (adjusted annually) regardless of the number of family members (at least two people) covered by the plan. If you are between the ages of 55 and 64, you can add an additional $1,000 annually. Couples in which both spouses are between ages of 55 and 64 can double this amount for up to an additional $2,000 a year.

So you have a group health plan? Great! However, if you are off work, how long can you continue your health coverage? When are the premium payments due at your employer? How much will the new monthly premiums be during the time you are separated without the employer contributions?

I recommend that you compare the costs of securing Private Portable Health Insurance coverage to the costs of available Employer Sponsored Group coverage if participation is not mandatory. In many cases, group coverage is not a bargain, for example, if the group overall has a high claim history and you do not. Ask a qualified agent to compare plans and shop for the best coverage for you. Know what is best for your financial situation and your coverage needs.

Are you without coverage now and believe you are uninsurable due to pre- existing conditions? Contact your state Insurance Commissioner to determine what your state guaranteed issue options are and then apply. These guaranteed issue plans may be expensive, and there may be some limits on coverage available. However, medical treatment without coverage will likely be much more expensive or even unobtainable without it. Why? Uninsured patients do not have the reduced negotiated rates the insured do. They pay full price.

Although there is still much turmoil on the subject, the Federal and State sponsored coverage exchanges could be explored.

If you are concerned about the possibility of an accident causing you to reach your high deductible quickly, and this holds you back from the higher deductible health insurance plan associated with an HSA or state pool, there may types of additional coverage you can consider. There are some remarkably low-cost plans available that pay benefits *only* for a true accidental medical or dental expense with maximum benefits usually ranging from $1,000 - $5,000 per occurrence. This type of plan complements your health insurance and is not a replacement for it. You need to do the math. Does the potential policy benefits warrant the premiums required for a policy that will pay for accidental medical or dental expenses only?

Step Two:
Free Prescription Medicine or Discount Drug Resources

USDiscountDrugCard.com

Take advantage of discounts and special savings on prescription medicine whether you have insurance coverage or not using a free discount drug program.

Go to the website and create a free ID card for each member of the family at http://www.usdiscountdrugcard.com/index.php .

You will receive your pre-activated personal discount prescription drug cards instantly from your computer printer using only your name; nothing else is required.

These cards are available absolutely free. If you lose your card, you can conveniently and quickly print another one. These free online discount drug cards are not insurance or insurance related. They can be used at over 50,000 pharmacies nationwide.

There is no income limits to be able to obtain a card, and no medical questions or other personal information is requested. The site has a link to locate a list of participating pharmacies in your area, and separate links to compare medication pricing among participating pharmacies.

If you do not have prescription coverage, or some drugs are excluded, this card can reduce your prescription costs up to 75%.

If you have private prescription coverage as a part of your existing plan, compare the cost of filling the prescription with your group or private insurance card, and this free discount card. You can fill the prescription with whichever is the lowest cost option.

Take into account your ongoing medication needs and determine if there is an advantage to having the costs of the prescription counted toward the deductible to your plan.

These free discount drug cards are not a replacement for health insurance. They are a complement to any other prescription coverage you currently have in place.

This free program is a good complement to Medicare part "D" plans during the dreaded "donut hole" period, or for non-covered meds.

BidRX.com

www.BidRX.com is an innovative internet based program for companies to save thousands of dollars on prescription medication for plan participants using a bidding system similar to Ebay. You can go to the site to see a quick demonstration.

This one of a kind, easy to use internet-based tool allows you to find the lowest cost provider for medications across the country with a few clicks of your mouse. You are no longer subject to the limited competition of the pharmacies in your local area.

The portal will allow you to see what other medication alternatives exist and instantly price compare.

There is a portal for your physician to use as well when they are seeking medication information and alternatives in this fast changing industry.

BidRX is set to launch an individual based portal for a very low monthly participation fee in February 2015.

PPARX

If you are in a financial crisis, there is another internet-based program you may want to look at: partnership For Prescription Assistance (PPARX). Their website is: https://www.pparx.org. Here you will find a resource that is income and need based.

Not all manufacturers participate but this does help many individuals secure needed medications for free or at a greatly reduced price. You must answer a few questions and it will give you a summary of the programs you may qualify for.

The US Discount Drug Card referenced above is part of the same discount drug card network that will appear on this site at the end of the process.

Step Three:
Health Savings Accounts and Employer Sponsored Pre-Tax Plans

If you choose an HSA, fund the tax-deductible HSA to the maximum allowed by law to have tax-free monies ready to pay medical expenses as you need them. This pre-planning saves you money by lowering your federal (and, if applicable, state) income tax bills.

What if you fund it and are blessed to remain healthy and never need the money during your working years? Great! When you get to retirement you will still have those dollars available to you for post-retirement medical expenses and they will be tax free along with any earnings that have accumulated.

If you use a group plan instead of an HSA, set aside the maximum out-of- pocket liability in a liquid account you can access if/when needed.

If your employer offers a pre-tax plan for non-covered medical expenses, learn how to use it. What is your annual maximum out of pocket limit on your health insurance for covered services (including deductibles and co-pays) in addition to your premiums? $2,000? $10,000? $20,000 or more?

How much is enough to set aside for next year's expected medical out of pocket expenses for your situation? Do not overfund this account.

In most cases you can only enroll and make changes once a year even if a qualifying life event occurs.

Consider the following normal medical expenses when making your contribution elections:

- Do you normally meet your deductible? How much is it?

- How much do you usually pay in co-pays after the deductible is met?

- What are your prescription costs monthly or annually?

- What are your eyeglasses or contact lens costs annually?

- Do you anticipate needing hearing aid batteries?

- What are your dental expenses for routine care and other needs?

- Will you be purchasing braces, crowns, dental implants or other expensive oral care services in the coming year?

- Do you participate in counseling sessions where you pay per service?

- What are your expected costs of acupuncture, chiropractic or other alternative eligible health care needs?

- Some individuals will also need to allow for long distance travel costs associated with treatment that must be provided out of the local area. This could include lodging and airline tickets.

Speak to your Human Resources department for a specific list of what medical related expenses you could have covered via your plan. They will also be able to inform you of any current or plan annual contribution limits.

Step Four:
Critical Illness and Key Man Critical Illness Insurance

A "Key Man" is an employee who is key to running your business. A lot of responsibility and profit can be generated by this person. You can have more than on "key Man" in a company.

Purchase a Critical Illness product that is triggered to pay a $10,000- $500,000 tax-free lump sum cash benefit upon any one of usually 20+ occurrences such as heart attack, stroke, cancer, blindness, etc. You generally choose the amount you would like to apply for.

The policy will go through underwriting, just like most other insurance coverage to determine if you qualify.

I suggest you apply to replace one to two years of wages. Within two years of the initial medical issue, there should be enough time to see what lifestyle changes need to be implemented by the household if the situation is permanent. Whether you will be cured or not, in all likelihood, at least at the two year mark, you should be able to go back to work in some capacity or know that in this case employment will never be likely again and plan your financial affairs accordingly.

A "critical illness only" policy is not a replacement for health or disability insurance. It is a complement to the health insurance and other disability coverage you already have in force.

Do you own a business? This type of policy can be used in a business arrangement to quickly infuse cash into your business in the event a business partner or a key employee has a disabling illness.

Why would your business want to pay for that kind of coverage? These funds can keep a business viable until the missing partner or key employee is able to return to full-time employment, or perhaps allow enough breathing room for the business to be sold to someone else instead of imploding.

You may want to have an agreement in place to continue pre-disability wages for a time for a partner before a buyout is triggered.

Remember, if you deduct the premiums as a business expense, then all the proceeds will be taxable income to the recipient. Talk to your accountant and tax professional about paying these business premiums with non-deductible dollars to enable proceeds to be tax free income when received.

If you would like assistance in this area, please contact me at this link for additional help:

http://www.amyroseherrick.pfyfn.com/request_quote

Step Five:
Long-Term Care and Disability Insurance

If you are age 55 and over, consider purchasing a Long-Term Care (LTC) policy that pays cash benefits if you become unable to care for yourself because of a loss of functional capacity or other cognitive loss such as Alzheimer's disease.

All or a portion of LTC premiums could be income-tax deductible if you meet tax guidelines.

Many states give tax breaks to residents who purchase LTC policies. Bring the amount you pay for premiums to the attention of your tax professional when you file your income taxes each year.

Younger workers should consider securing an Individual Disability plan to provide a disability income stream. Depending on your age or occupation, benefits may be payable to age 65.

Individual disability premiums are not tax deductible. That also means the proceeds are not taxable income when received.

You may be able to secure either LTC or disability coverage via your employer. Read the coverage parameters carefully. Not all plans are portable. This means that when you leave your employer, or if they decide to terminate the plan, you cannot continue the coverage as an individual policy. If you have a pre-existing condition, securing replacement coverage may not be possible when an old policy is terminated or allowed to lapse.

Many employer-sponsored disability plans favor low wage earners with short periods of income replacement of up to 70% of wages during a loss (for example: a $2,000 maximum benefit per month, which is only payable for six months). The same group policy may not be an adequate short-term monthly benefit for the higher wage earners in the same company because the maximum policy limits might only replace a smaller fraction of their earnings.

It is possible to have great or even excellent short-term coverage at work and very bad or poor long-term coverage (or vice versa).

High wage earners may need to have at least two coordinated policies in place to replace between 60% and 70% of their income, and most insurers limit policy maximum coverage liability to $7,000 - $10,000 per person, per month. A high wage individual may need to implement a combination of disability and LTC policies.

How much is enough coverage for either LTC or Disability insurance? An experienced agent will examine each individual situation, taking into account existing employer sponsored options, cash resources, occupation, age and your preferences in order to design your coverage package.

Another innovation that has entered the marketplace from a few insurers is a combination policy that provides life insurance and the advancement of death benefits in the same policy for a qualified illness. Whether you access all the proceeds for a qualified illness, death or any combination of the two, the policy pays the face amount in benefits. If you cancel the policy and have not received benefits, unless you have designed it to build cash value in addition to providing benefits, it will have little or no cash accumulated at the time it is terminated.

Other combination policies provide for a one time lump sum deposit that is multiplied for Long Term Care Events if they occur, has a larger than the amount deposited in a death benefit from the moment of issue. A separate component of the policy has a refund provision allowing you to receive all of your deposit back at any time when cancelling the policy. Some combination policies have a short period from inception deducting a small percentage penalty if you cancelled the policy in the first three to five years; after that, you would receive a full refund.

In cancellation situations, there could be a 1099 issued. Why? You would need to have the cost of the benefit for Long Term Care included in your income if the policy is cancelled before either the death benefit or the long Term care benefits were paid.

It's all about options!

If you would like assistance in this area, please contact me for a quote:

http://www.amyroseherrick.pfyfn.com/request_quote

Step Six:
Your Crisis Cash Plan

Set aside an emergency cash cushion at least equal to the elimination period on your LTC or disability plan before anticipated income streams are activated.

Some creative ways to help reach this goal until you build the actual cash reserve amount include:

• Earmark a portion of cash values in permanent life insurance. You could loan money from the policy at a low interest rate that may never need to be repaid.

• Your ROTH IRA contributions (not earnings) could be a tax free source of income at any age.

• Earmark an investment account to be liquidated.

• Identify in advance assets that can be sold quickly.

• Know in advance where the short-term funds will be coming from during a crisis.

Make sure your most likely caregivers or the person with your Power of Attorney (POA) also knows your plan.

Small business owners and the self-employed need to identify or set aside additional working capital resources or lines of credit. This allows their businesses to continue operations with a minimum of interruption of day to day operations.

Step Seven:
Secure Air Ambulance Coverage

One area that has changed dramatically in recent years due to technology advances in the medical care delivery field is the use of air ambulance services. Helicopter pads on top of our medical facilities have become increasingly common. These lifesaving helicopters are specially equipped and staffed with strategically trained paramedics, doctors and nurses and transport the emergency patient quickly to a facility that can provide more advanced care much faster than ground transportation.

If you travel frequently for business or pleasure, enjoy remote locations, cruise often, scuba dive, hike, motor home, have young accident prone children or spouses, vacation or live abroad part of the year, or plan to, this is certainly a product you need to explore.

Chapter Three:
Insurance Products

I have examined and recommended many instances in which the costs of group health insurance premiums alone are more than the cost of a non-work sponsored income and asset protection strategy secured on an individual basis.

This type of a total income and asset protection approach is a great idea to take to your Human Resources department as a potential alternative to the traditional in-force group low-deductible policy arrangements. These types of non-traditional comprehensive approaches can be extremely effective when a business is attempting to improve coverage options to attract or retain key employees.

In many cases, these types of coordinated plans are used as a means to control the double-digit spiraling benefit costs businesses are faced with on traditional plans.

Disability Income Replacement Insurance Overview

Employer sponsored coverage

This is often the easiest coverage to qualify for in a group setting.

This benefit normally replaces about 60% of your pre-tax earnings.

Read and understand the policy fine print.

The plan may only be based on your base wages and specifically exclude bonuses.

The plan may have a monthly maximum that covers support staff but is inadequate for executive level positions standing alone.

The employer owns the group policy and you are allowed to participate in the plan as an individual only as long as you are an employee at the company.

The premiums are deducted from payroll with your authorization.

Benefits can be short term only or long term only or a combination of the two coverages in separate policies.

Short term coverage may be for no more than six months of benefits after a short waiting or elimination period of perhaps 7 to14 days.

Long term coverage may pay benefits if you are eligible up to age 65 or a set number of years after a longer waiting period of perhaps 90 days, 180 days or one year.

If the premiums are deducted from payroll on a pre-tax basis, you will save a few dollars in income taxes today, but every dollar of benefits will be taxable income to you later. Keep in mind the income tax load incurred on taxable disability benefits when distributed further erodes your actual net income received.

I suggest you always pay group plans with after-tax dollars whenever possible. Just one month of drawing taxable disability benefits incurring income taxes could quickly erase years of tiny annual prior income tax savings for you. Every one of those future checks would be taxable going forward too. Income taxes are even more expensive when you have less to pay for them.

You also need to know if the coverage is portable or has any conversion options. This feature allows you to take the policy with you if you left the employer by changing the policy over to individual coverage (usually within a short 30 day window of separation).

Privately purchased coverage

This requires a formal application and full underwriting by an insurance company before you are offered coverage.

If you have a pre-existing condition the insurance company may offer coverage with an exclusion rider. If this occurs everything else would be covered except the specified excluded illness or condition.

When exclusion is a part of a policy, ask when you could reapply for a review to have the exclusion removed. This could be in six months, a year or some other time frame. Follow up promptly as soon as possible based on the time frame until you can get the exclusion removed. You will not have to pay for this request to review your exclusion but you may be required to submit to a new para-med examination.

Private policy benefits normally replace about 60% of your pre-tax earnings.

If you are a high wage earner you may have to coordinate coverage from multiple insurers. Why? Many insurers who offer this product limit their exposure by having a limit of $5,000 to $10,000 a month disability income coverage maximum per person.

The premiums are paid annually or by monthly bank drafts on your checking account with your authorization.

Long term coverage may pay benefits if you are eligible up to age 65 or a set number of years after a longer waiting period of perhaps 60 days, 90 days, 180 days or one year.

Premiums are always paid in individually owned policies after tax making any private disability benefits nontaxable income to you when received.

Long-Term Care Insurance Overview

The American Association for Long Term Care Insurance reported in 2012 that the largest open claim, filed by a woman who has been receiving benefits under her policy for 15 years, had reached $1.7 million in benefits and was still paying her for the lifetime benefits she purchased in her policy.

The same report detailed that more than two thirds of new claimants for policy benefits in 2011 were women.

Women generally have longer life expectancies than men.

Here are some current statistics on how long term care is actually used based on insured claims during 2014 at Genworth Financial, a well-known long term care policy provider:

- Youngest claimant was only 27 years old.

- Oldest claimant was 103 years old.

- Most expensive claim for lifetime benefits Genworth has paid out has been $1,300,000+ (to date, ongoing).

- 15% of claims lasted more than 5 years.

- If a claim lasted more than one year, it lasted on average 3.9 years.

- 50% of claims have lasted more than a year.

- 71% of claims started with home health care benefits being used first.

- Only 13% of the claims started in an assisted living facility.

- 16% of claims started at the nursing home level.

Note that the majority of claims started with home health care at 71%. This means the policy home health care components are vital to an individual's ability to maintain an independent living status outside of a nursing home or assisted living facility for as long as possible. Failure to include home health care benefits in your LTC policy would limit the insured's choices for financial assistance for a qualifying event when care dollars are most needed.

The same 2014 Genworth report dispelled the myth that claims only happen at "older" ages. A little over 1 in 10 claims were for individuals under the age of 69.

- .3% of claimants were younger than age 50.

- 1.9% were ages 50-59.

- 8.7% were aged 60-69.

- 25.4% were ages 70-79.

• 63.7% were past the age of 80.

The good news is we are living longer than prior generations! If you were born just 100 years ago, your life expectancy was only an average age of 47. A female child born today has a life expectancy of just over 81 years. Males have a life expectancy of just over 76 years.

With that good news, comes some sobering news. According to a report released by ACLI in November 2014, 70% of those who are currently age 65 will require long term care in their lifetimes.

If you are planning to max out your 401(k) or have the house paid off before age 65 it probably won't be sufficient LTC funding planning. Only a fraction of the identified "at risk" 70% of the 65+ population expected to incur LTC expenses has taken any action to secure LTC insurance. The majority of those in the age bracket of 45 to 64 have not factored this potentially huge liability into their financial plans either before or after retirement.

The number one objection to buying LTC or a combination policy with life insurance benefits is the argument that it costs too much. The key to affording peace of mind is to design a plan that complements other resources you already have in place.

Types of LTC Coverage

You may or may not have access to this coverage through your employer as a group benefit.

Traditional Reimbursement Plan

A traditional reimbursement plan pays much like your health insurance.

You should be warned that someone must devote a lot of time keeping track of every medical-related expense, and that person must also be diligent in submitting each and every day's worth of costs for consideration and reimbursement.

Some exhausted family members say that managing care giving, submission of claims to all involved insurers, and management of payments for all the services provided is more than a full-time job and requires spreadsheets just to keep track of all the paperwork required.

Cash Benefit Plan

This type of plan pays cash benefits if you cannot perform two "Adult Daily Living" activities (ADLs).

This type of plan is much simpler to deal with than the Traditional Reimburse Plan because you don't need to document how you are spending the money.

A check simply arrives once a month after the patient has been qualified for benefits.

This type of policy dramatically lessens the headaches, time, and bookkeeping burden on caregivers by eliminating the need to keep track of the submissions, reimbursement, payment and reconciliation steps.

Combination Life and Long Term Care Alternative Plan

This plan is a life insurance policy that also pays a death benefit.

It might include long term care alternative life insurance advancement features of either a traditional reimbursement plan or a cash benefit plan.

Policy provisions vary between insurers and products approved for sale offered in your jurisdiction.

In these policies death benefits are either advanced or a separate rider provides the long term care alternative benefits to the family member.

Applicants must meet insurability guidelines to secure this kind of coverage.

Combination Annuity and Long Term Care Alternative Plan

This alternative is an annuity policy sold by an insurance company invested with the intent to grow the principal for later use.

The underlying annuity could be a fixed rate or variable product invested in a combination of stocks, bonds or fixed accounts.

Policy provisions will vary between insurers and products approved for sale and offered in your jurisdiction.

These policies can be structured to provide a lifetime income that is doubled for long term care qualified events.

Even if the amount of principal and any earnings invested is exhausted and the contract has no value left in it, the monthly benefits continue for the annuitant's lifetime.

Generally, there is little or very limited medical underwriting for this feature.

Critical Illness Coverage Overview

This unique insurance product that was created in the 1990's as an answer to the spiraling costs of medical care.

This coverage provides a lump-sum, tax-free payment should a policyholder suffer from certain specific critical conditions.

This policy is usually written for a lump sum face amount of $10,000 - $1,000,000 per insured.

The proceeds are tax free to spend however you chose.

The top three common conditions that might trigger a lump sum payment include cancer, heart attack, and stroke.

Many policies cover several other conditions including kidney/renal failure, paralysis, and blindness.

There are a few products available for purchase that can add a critical illness rider on your life insurance policy at the time of purchase, or as an advancement of a portion of the policy death benefits if you do not secure a critical illness only policy.

Air Ambulance Coverage Overview

This service is not always covered in many health insurance policies. If it is included, there may be a low limit of actual dollar reimbursement per flight or your coverage may be available only in a limited local service area.

In most cases any foreign travel or out of network providers are completely excluded from coverage. If there is out of area coverage in the policy, using out of network providers generally carries much higher deductibles if covered at all.

All unpaid air ambulance services provided leave the patient with substantial out of pocket costs to bear after any insurance proceeds if any were applied.

Costs for medical air flight can be as low as $10,000 for a short trip to well over $50,000 or more depending on the duration and location of the flight needed.

Example one: You are in the middle of the Caribbean on a tiny island enjoying a long planned vacation when you have a sudden onset of a debilitating headache that is quickly diagnosed as an aneurysm. You need to be transported to the closest qualified trauma center in Miami for immediate emergency care; your survival depends on this. How will your family arrange to get you a flight and then pay for that emergency medical air flight to save your life before liftoff occurs?

Example two: You are traveling across the US in your motor home. You stop at one of our beautiful remote natural parks. You have a heart attack and the closest cardiac center is over 200 hundred rugged miles away and the ambulance still needs to get here from the closest town. You leave the motor home behind as your spouse travels with you. Who will drive that motor home back home for you? Who will pay for the air flight you so desperately need and the travel back home where you will recuperate before getting back on the road again?

You can secure single or family air ambulance coverage for a fraction of the cost of one covered event.

You can choose a policy with a limited coverage area or you can purchase a policy to cover you wherever you are in the U.S. or worldwide.

This coverage is an essential insurance to have for those who travel on business or pleasure, extended motor home trips, live in remote areas or plan to travel abroad.

If you live on an island as I do such as St Croix in the US Virgin Islands, air ambulance coverage is a lifesaving essential part of our overall healthcare delivery system for those who purchase it.

What exactly is an air ambulance?

When a ground ambulance can't get to your location, or get you to an emergency center fast enough, an air ambulance is called in for rescue and transport. Air ambulances are also used in metro areas when time to do ground transportation to a trauma center would take too long.

Air ambulances are state-of-the-art flying aviation based medical miracles when it comes to saving lives. They are specially equipped and staffed by highly trained paramedics, emergency medical technicians and sometimes have on board doctors and nurses.

What does air ambulance insurance typically cover?

Speak to your agent to find out what coverage your policy provides. Common examples of coverage include:

- Assistance in arranging emergency care from facility to facility

- Air fares back home for you and traveling companion or to return minor age children home

- Air flight Medical care you require during transportation such as oxygen or life support

- Transportation to and from the aircraft ("bedside to bedside" service)

- The delivery of a motor home back to your residence if you were air lifted out when more than 100 miles away from home

- Transportation of the remains to your funeral home of choice if you do not survive

- 24/7/365 assistance is a phone call away

- Other benefits

Be aware that in some policies you may only be covered for life flights abroad if you notify them in advance of your planned travel. It is usually as easy as a quick call to an 800 number.

Chapter Four:
Health Care Sharing Ministry Alternatives

What is Health Care Sharing?

First and foremost understand this is not health insurance. This program is not, will not and is never intended to operate like an insurance company.

The health care sharing concept is a Biblical based approach to paying for health care of the members based on Biblical passages applied to medical costs today for singles and families sharing a same faith based belief on medical care costs.

This program is not and will not be a good fit for those who do not share the same faith based values. The program is based on established Biblical principles and as a result there are lifestyle choices that are not covered, supported or encouraged.

I am including this little known resource as an alternative designed to help a variety of readers and their families.

Samaritan Ministries

First you need to understand what a "Share" consists of. Each member of the plan consistently remits a pre-established "Share" amount each month.

The Samaritan ministries program's website is located at **http://samaritanministries.org**.

According to the website, "shares" are sent directly through the mail to members with "needs."

Samaritan Ministries uses a database that randomly matches "shares" with "needs" so that the sharing is coordinated.

Samaritan Ministries' information on the website reports that it publishes a monthly newsletter mailing that reports the total "shares" and "needs". They include an individualized Share Notice for each member household. The Share Notice tells each household how to pray for a specific member with a "need" and what his/her address is, so the "share" can be sent to him/her.

I was surprised to learn that in a typical month less than 10% of the members are experiencing a "need."

Medical costs and providers are not handled like a PPO or other In/Out of Network type service area restrictions you may be used to. Remember, this is not insurance.

A member receives health care treatment from a provider of his/her choice. Members are responsible for collecting and forwarding the bills to Samaritan Ministries. Samaritan Ministries will look over the submissions to verify that the "need" and the bills presented meet the medi-share program guidelines.

As of 2/2015 the website reported they had over 40,000 member households participating in the ministry. At that time there was about $10 million available each month to meet health care "needs" from the "shares" remitted by the member households.

You should consult the Samaritans Ministries website for more information.

Christian Care Ministry

Another medi-share program was developed by Christian Care Ministry. Their website is https://mychristiancare.org.

Christian Care Ministry is different in that their model is designed to work with the members' providers to submit bills directly to Christian Care Ministry for processing and discounting. They will also handle payment to the providers. Consult the website for specific details.

Comparison

I was able to find this helpful chart to help you compare the two different plans mentioned for reference at http://www.garynorth.com/Opt-Out.pdf.

Review the information contained on the different websites and call the number listed for specific questions.

Health Care Exemption Eligible

Although the heath care climate is ever changing, as of 2/2015 both of these programs are exempt from what has been nicknamed the "Obamacare" mandates.

Chapter Five:
Important Documents

Document One: Financial Power of Attorney

You need to have this important document in place so that pending personal and business issues can continue without you through your representative.

I suggest you go three levels deep naming your chosen representatives on these types of documents. Make your first choice, and then select a second choice, and even a third choice, in case the preferred person cannot serve in that capacity at the time you really need them.

Make sure copies are in the possession of all the persons listed.

Be specific. Do not list "my brother Bill Smith". Include full names, address, work, cell and home phone numbers, email addresses, any and all ways these people could be contacted quickly in an emergency. This also makes the identity of these people easily verifiable.

Document Two: Living Will or Medical Directive

What do you want to happen to you in a medical crisis?

If you want an armed guard to keep family members away from your ventilator electrical cord, and want every known method known to medical science applied to keep you alive, put it in print! On the other hand, if you desire no heroic efforts, or for religious reasons you do not want blood transfusions, or you desire that your organs, skin, bones or any other part of your body are to be used for transplants or medical science, write it down.

Do not simply tell someone what you want and assume they will be able to honor your wishes in times of crisis. Write it down and pass out copies!

Resign and redate them at least once a year to keep your wishes current as your health changes.

Document Three: Medical Power of Attorney

You need to have this important document in place so that a person you trust can step in to make your medical treatment decisions when you are unable to do so due to illness or injury.

This may or may not be the same person as your Financial Power of Attorney. These are separate documents.

I suggest you go three levels deep naming your chosen representatives on these types of documents. Make your first choice, and then select a second choice, and even a third choice, in case the preferred person cannot serve in that capacity at the time you really need them.

Make sure copies are in the possession of all the persons listed.

Be specific. Do not list "my sister Sarah Jones." Include full names, address, work, cell and home phone numbers, email addresses, any and all ways these people could be contacted quickly in an emergency. This also makes the identity of these people easily verifiable.

Document Four: Updated Will

If you do not recover, do not leave an additional mess of an estate that has to be sorted out and settled based on existing state or residential jurisdiction laws to your grieving survivors.

Do potential executors have copies, know where it is stored for easy retrieval or is this very important document hidden somewhere that no one besides you will find it? For example, a safety deposit box only in your name is not easily accessible to your family when you are deceased. Make it easy for your loved ones to find it and be able to access it.

Document Five: List of Insurance Policies and Coverage

Make sure you include all of your policy numbers and the contact numbers for the insurance companies.

In the event of an emergency, a spouse or other representative may need to refer and activate many plans in a timely manner or you may lose the benefits you earned and paid for.

Include life, health and accident plans, group coverage, disability policies, LTC, Air Ambulance, etc.

Pass out copies of this important list to your POA!

Document Six: "The Family Love Letter"

"The Family Love Letter" is a wonderful well thought out 40-plus page booklet I often use with my clients. I highly recommend it.

This excellent online resource for family members of any asset level allows you to easily compile, all your important household financial information including: your assets, important contact information for advisors, insurance information, medical wishes, funeral instructions, account passwords, other key financial data, estate information and more - all in one convenient place.

This easy-to-complete and thorough resource booklet can be ordered for just a few dollars.

If you have ever had to settle an estate in array while grieving, or step in to manage the finances of a loved one whose affairs you know little or nothing about, you will appreciate how valuable this tool is.

This booklet is truly a practical, lasting love letter to your family. Order one for every family member. Here is a helpful link: http://www.familyloveletter.com .

Chapter Six:
Special Considerations

Physically and Developmentally Disabled Family Members

In many families, one person coordinates the ongoing care of a child or adult with disabilities.

In these cases, the primary caregiver needs to leave information and instructions for their replacement during a caregiver's medical crisis or death.

Identify who will be responsible for the disabled family member if the current primary care person is no longer able to do so. Speak frankly to anyone you consider for this responsibility to determine if they are willing and able to take over this responsibility. It is better for someone to be honest and say "no" now if they cannot handle this challenge rather than later.

Secure at least three different possible alternate caregivers so your loved one is never in the hands of the courts looking for a care solution.

Compile a Letter of Intent that is coordinated with a future guardian the event someone else must fill in for you at the primary caregiver.

Draft a guide for your replacement including everything what a future guardian needs to know to the situation with a minimum of stress on everyone involved. Specify the following: the exact diagnosis or condition, what testing has been done, where the medical records are located, the local pharmacy number, regularly scheduled activities, insurance information, and the patient's likes, dislikes, allergies, and medication schedules. It would also be very helpful to include names and numbers of any respite care providers you have used in the past who know your situation and would be good resource to call for help in a crisis.

If you are not a writer or good typist, then use an unlimited dictation service for a month and dictate it! The dictations will come back by email and can be compiled and edits for a very low cost. One service I would suggest for this is Copytalk. You can visit their website at https://www.copytalk.com/ct/ for more information. I would suggest you spell and repeat the spelling of any difficult words such as medication spellings, specific medical condition terminologies or other unusual spellings.

If you have not already done so, set up a Special Needs Trust to provide a safety net beyond Social Security and Medicaid for this special family member. If you are not familiar with these types of planning tools, Special Needs Trusts (when properly designed) will not count as an available resource when it comes time to determine eligibility for any type of government-sponsored financial aid.

Once the trust is in place, you should make it a priority to update all or a portion of your beneficiary designations on your retirement accounts, company benefits, and life insurance policies naming the trust (NOT the disabled family member) as the beneficiary. Other family members may contribute to this trust if desired.

Warning! Talk to your attorney and tax person for assistance before naming the trust as beneficiary on those types of accounts so you clearly understand the potential tax consequences of doing so.

A frequent alternative to a trust arrangement used for disabled family members is to use annuity products with restricted beneficiaries so that they only have lifetime benefits in installments in a frequency of your choosing but not direct access to the principal only. This payout restriction to named beneficiaries can only be changed by the annuity owner and is triggered at the annuity owner's death. It is revocable at any time prior to death unless you make it irrevocable at inception.

In most jurisdictions, if your loved one has as little as $2,000 in some in his or her name, he or she will not be ineligible to receive any benefits until the assets are exhausted and what has been spent on his or her care has been documented. This is likely not the scenario you had in mind. Any proceeds left in the trust or in the restricted annuity payment arrangement at the patient's death are assigned to the beneficiaries listed in the trust documents or annuity beneficiary records.

It is common to distribute unused trust assets to other family members or a favorite charity after the death of the disabled loved one when the trust is no longer needed.

Have you established legal guardianship?

Parents won't have an automatic say about the care of a minor child, or access to medical records after he or she turns 18. By retaining legal guardianship of a disabled family member of any age, families can put in place tools such as trusts and limited access to bank accounts and investments to protect loved ones from people who don't have his or her best interests at heart and intend to defraud the patient of his or her assets.

Health insurance continuation after the retirement or death of the primary policyholder must be planned in advance. In most cases, a disabled minor child is covered under his or her parent or guardian's group health insurance plan until the parent or guardian is no longer employed with that company if the disability occurred before the 22nd birthday. Let your human resources officer and the insurance companies know which insured is disabled to make sure he or she remains covered.

If the child risks loss of coverage because of a separation, know in advance what other options need to be applied for and secured within 30 days of separation so there is no gap in coverage.

Remember to contact your State Insurance Commissioner for information about guaranteed insurability options in your state and assistance in complex situations so you know which laws and rules apply.

Documents should be distributed to key family members, physicians, trust officers and anyone else who may be called on in an emergency to help with a guardian transition.

Have you secured an attorney?

You must also involve a competent, caring attorney in your family affairs.

This is not a luxury; it is a necessity.

You will also need to revisit your documents from time to time and update them in the event laws and circumstances change.

Cohabitating Households

For the first time in census history, married couples account for the minority of households. In the 2010 Census only 48% of households were married couples.

This group is probably the least protected medically and financially in the event of a separation, medical crisis or death.

Who are some common examples of cohabitating households?

- Young adults living with grandparents or other relatives while attending school

- Adult roommates

- Opposite sex couples

- Same sex couples

Any rights you desire need to be created using legal documents. The most common of these include wills, living wills, advance medical directives including what non-family members can visit you, a domestic partner agreement, parenting agreement, revocable living trusts, life insurance trusts, and durable powers of attorney for finances.

Child Trends Data Bank helps us see the changing demographics of childbirth and resulting challenges this creates:

Younger women are substantially more likely than older women to have a child outside of marriage.

In 2004, the most recent year for which data by all ages are available, the overwhelming majority of teenage births were to unmarried young women (97.4% for teens under age 15 and 82.4% for 15 to 19 year olds), compared with slightly over half of births to women ages 20 to 24 (54.8%), over one-quarter of births to women ages 25 to 29 (27.8%), and 15 to 16% of births to women in their 30s.

Has paternity been firmly established?

What about any future Social Security benefits for any children born outside of marriage? This is a critical consideration for a surviving parent in the event the custodial parent disabled and/or dies without establishing paternity on his child.

What about health insurance for children of non-married partners? Is the coverage work related and is it convertible to individual policies? If so, what is the time frame to convert after the disability or death of the other partner?

Have you reviewed your investment accounts, credit cards, bank accounts and credit lines? Do you have any of these titled together? Are you a joint holder or a single user? What will be your future limits of access to cash assets? What is your possible financial liability for the balances owed?

Building Your Financial Team

If you really want to protect your partner and children, you need to take responsible action now. How? You need to build a team consisting of a qualified attorney and a qualified financial professional to design and assist you in implementing a complete package of medical/legal planning for your non-traditional family.

After you have this package completed, update it periodically to insure that it remains current.

Any issue that is not addressed in a valid legal document is an issue that is in jeopardy of physically, emotionally and financially harming your partner or children at the time of your death or disability.

Conclusion:
Getting Started

Are you hesitating for financial reasons?

The worst excuse is, "I can't afford it".

You may be closer to the edge of financial disaster from a medical cause than you may be willing to admit.

You could be poised to lose everything in a short period of time because of procrastination or denial.

Perhaps you are concerned about the time and energy it will take you and others to implement changes.

Are you prepared to face the possibility that you or a family member may become disabled, and/or never fully recover from an unexpected birth defect, accident or illness?

Yes, it can be frightening to consider scenarios involving your potential disability or death, but with support from family and friends you can all get through it without becoming financially devastated.

You and your family have everything to lose and nothing to gain doing nothing. Now you know what to do!

The next section is a short checklist of the items discussed in this book you may need to secure or explore in more depth.

Suggested Coverages and Important Documents Checklist

	Need	Have	Copies given to POA
—Chapter Two: Seven Steps to Take to Protect Your Family Assets			
Health Insurance	____	____	____
USDiscountDrugCard.com	____	____	____
BidRX.com	____	____	____
PPARX.org	____	____	____
H.S.A. or Employer Flexible Spending Account	____	____	
—Chapter Three: Insurance Products			
Disability Insurance	____	____	
Employer Sponsored Short Term	____	____	
Employer Sponsored Long Term	____	____	
Private Short Term	____	____	
Private Long Term	____	____	
Long Term Care Insurance	____	____	
Employer sponsored	____	____	
Private	____	____	
Tax Free Lump Sum Critical Illness Insurance	____	____	
Individual	____	____	
Key Man Coverage for the Business	____	____	
Air Ambulance Coverage	____	____	
List of all insurance policies and phone numbers	____	____	____

—Chapter Four: Health Care Sharing Ministry Alternatives

	Need	Have	Copies given to POA
Medi-Share Health Insurance Alternatives Samaritan ministries International	____	____	____
My Christian Care	____	____	____
Crisis cash plan for $_____	____	____	____

—Chapter Five: Important Documents

	Need	Have	Copies given to POA
Will	____	____	____
Living Will or Medical Directive	____	____	____
Financial Power of Attorney	____	____	____
Medical Power of Attorney	____	____	____
Family Love Letter	____	____	____

http://www.familyloveletter.com

—Chapter Six: Special Considerations for Special Needs Family Members

	Need	Have	Copies given to POA
Letter of Instruction	____	____	____
List of all current medications	____	____	____
Medical Diagnosis	____	____	____
Respite Contacts	____	____	____
List of Known Allergies	____	____	____
Daily Schedule	____	____	____
Likes and Dislikes	____	____	____
Guardianship Established	____	____	____
POA Established for this person	____	____	____

Special Needs Trust   ____ ____   ____

Family Attorney   ____ ____   ____

About the Author

Amy Rose Herrick launched Money With Amy in late 2014 to enable her to share her wisdom and expertise acquired in her 30-plus years of experience in the financial services field.

She is a Chartered Financial Consultant (ChFC).

Beginning in 1991 she expanded her professional expertise and ongoing licensing to include earning the title of Insurance Agent for Life, Disability, Critical Illness, Long Term Care and Air Ambulance coverages.

During the same time she completed a career change from corporate clients to exclusively serving the needs of individual and a small business based clientele.

Not satisfied that she had all the planning tools needed to advise clients to the best of her ability in changing economic climates, in the early 90's she took the necessary training and ongoing educational hours necessary to secure her ability as a tax professional too.

Her articles have appeared in numerous publications. Amy accepted short term assignments for regular newspaper columns on specific items of public interest now and then in addition to her private practice demands. She was selected to contribute two chapters to books that were collaborative efforts between multiple professionals in 2007 and 2010.

In addition to her writing and other business activities, Amy is a dynamic public speaker who is able to engage with her audiences by breaking down complex concepts into manageable ideas that are easily understood using custom designed presentations.

Amy's planning expertise extends into situations that encompass corporate, individual and small business financial issues related to cash flow, debt structure, income tax reduction, charitable giving, business succession plans, mental or physical incapacity at any age, Life Insurance Settlements for unwanted policies and overall estate planning.

Amy and her family relocated from the Midwest to call the beautiful island of St. Croix their family home in early 2011.

Amy continues to serve a wide range of clients on the U.S. mainland coast to coast as well as clients residing in the US Virgin Islands.

In her free time she enjoys traveling, photography and she has a flair for art.

For Additional Information

Info@MoneyWithAmy.com

Follow Amy on Facebook

https://www.facebook.com/moneywithamy

Visit our website

www.MoneyWithAmy.com

Books by Amy Rose Herrick

Knowing Your Life Partner- 25 Questions to ask and answer before making a commitment

Family Medical Planning

Small Business Ownership Financial Mistakes

Life Planning - Living Together Physically and Financially

British Virgin Islands Short Sailing Trip Hai Ku Impressions with Photographs

25 Questions to Ask Before Remarriage

Marriage After Retirement 25 Questions to Ask